MEDICAL MICROBIOLOGY

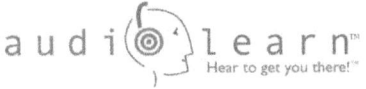

Table of Contents

i

Microbiology

Microbiology is the study of very small living creatures, often referred to as microorganisms. They include viruses, bacteria and fungi. The study of these microorganisms is significant and medically relevant because of frequent microbial diseases that can be severe and sometimes deadly to humans.

This audiobook will provide a detailed list and description of all medically significant viruses, bacteria and fungi.

Viruses

Viruses are the smallest of the microorganisms that we will review in this audiobook.

To reproduce viruses must infect other living cells. They are spread through the air. There are two classes of viruses: either DNA or RNA.

Influenza Virus

The *Influenza virus* is the cause of the common flu. Complications of the flu can result in Pneumonia in senior citizens and Reyes Syndrome in children that take aspirin.

The Influenza Virus is a negative single stranded RNA Orthomyxo */Or' tho mik' so/* Virus.

The Influenza Virus expresses potential virulence factors including Hemagglutinin (HA) glycoprotein that binds to the red blood cells. It can also bind to receptors on the cells of the upper respiratory tract that can result in viral RNA being dumped into these cells. The Influenza Virus also can cause Neurominidase (NA) glycoprotein, which is a breaking down of Neuraminic Acid.

The Influenza Virus can be treated with Amantadine. It can be prevented with a vaccine that prevents upcoating of Influenza Type A.

Parainfluenza Virus

The *Parainfluenza Virus* can cause upper respiratory infections in adults, such as, Bronchitis, Pharyngitis and Rhinitis. It is also the common cause of Viral Pneumonia and Croup in children.

The Parainfluenza Virus is a negative single stranded RNA Paramyxo */peramik' so/* Virus.

The Parainfluenza Virus expresses potential virulence factors including glycoproteins with combined HA and NA activity and F-Protein that results in multinucleated giant cells.

The Parainfluenza Virus is treated with supportive care.

Respiratory Syncytial Virus

The Respiratory Syncytial Virus is the most common cause of pneumonia in infants under six months of age.

The Respiratory Syncytial Virus is a negative single stranded RNA Paramyxo */peramik' so/* Virus.

The Respiratory Syncital Virus expresses potential virulence factors including F-Protein and no HA or NA glycoproteins.

The Respiratory Syncytial Virus is treated with supportive care and Ribavirin.

Mumps Virus

The Mumps Virus causes painful swelling of the Parotid Gland and very painful testicular inflammation. It can also cause Meningitis and Encephalitis.

4

The Mumps Virus is a negative single stranded RNA Paramyxo /peramik' so/ Virus.

The Mumps Virus expresses potential virulence factors including glycoproteins with combined HA and NA activity and F-protein.

The MMR (Measles, Mumps, Rubella) Vaccine prevents the Mumps Virus.

Measles Virus

The Measles (Rubeola) Virus causes protodome, small red based blue-white centered lesions in the mouth, and a rash from head to toe. Complications of the measles virus include pneumonia, eye damage, Encephalitis and a risk of fetal death if acquired by a woman in the first trimester of pregnancy.

The Measles Virus is a negative single stranded RNA Paramyxo /peramik' so/ Virus.

The Measles Virus expresses potential virulence factors including HA and F-protein.

The Measles Virus can also be prevented by the MMR (Measles, Mumps, Rubella Vaccine.

Hepatitis A Virus

The Hepatitis A Virus causes Acute Viral Hepatitis with fever, jaundice, and an enlarged liver. This condition never becomes chronic.

The Hepatitis A Virus is a positive single-stranded RNA

Picorna /pe-kor' na/ Viridae /vir' ide/ Virus.

Hepatitis A is transmitted via feces or orally.

Hepatitis A is treated with a pooled immune serum globulin and supportive care. Hepatitis A can be prevented with the Hepatitis A Vaccination.

Hepatitis B Virus

The Hepatitis B Virus causes Acute Viral Hepatitis and Fulminant Hepatitis, which is a Severe Acute Hepatitis that causes rapid destruction of the liver. Complications of Hepatitis B include Primary Hepatocellular Carcinoma and Cirrhosis of the liver.

The Hepatitis B Virus is a double-stranded DNA Hepadna /hep' adna/ Viridae /vir' ide/ Virus.

Hepatitis B is transmitted via blood transfusions contaminated needle sticks, sexually and through the placenta.

Hepatitis B is prevented with a Hepatitis B Vaccine that is now given to all infants at birth. The Hepatitis B Virus is treated with Alpha-Interferon Lamivudine.

Hepatitis C Virus

The Hepatitis C Virus causes Acute Viral Hepatitis. 50% of those infected will get Chronic Hepatitis and 20% will develop Cirrhosis of the liver. Contracting Hepatitis C also increases the risk of developing primary Hepatocellular Carcinoma.

The Hepatitis C Virus is a single-stranded RNA Flavivirus

/fla' vi' vi' rus/.

Hepatitis C is transmitted via blood transfusions contaminated needle sticks, sexually and through the placenta.

The treatment for Hepatitis C is Alpha-Interferon Ribavirin.

Hepatitis D Virus

The Hepatitis D Virus is acquired as a co-infection with Hepatitis B and can cause Acute Hepatitis. Complications of Hepatitis D include Fulminant Hepatitis and Cirrhosis of the liver.

The Hepatitis D Virus is an incomplete RNA Virus. It can only infect with the assistance of the Hepatitis B Virus.

Hepatitis D is transmitted via blood transfusions infected needle sticks, sexually and through the placenta.

The only way to control the Hepatitis D virus is to control the Hepatitis B infection from spreading by vaccination.

Hepatitis E Virus

The Hepatitis E Virus causes Acute Viral Hepatitis, which includes fever, jaundice, and a painful enlarged liver. This strain of Hepatitis is responsible for epidemics in Asia, but is very rare in the United States.

The Hepatitis E Virus is a single stranded RNA Calicivirus */kalis' i vi' rus/.*

Hepatitis E is transmitted via feces or orally.

There is no treatment for Hepatitis E.

Hepatitis G Virus

The Hepatitis G Virus has not been conclusively shown to cause liver disease.

The Hepatitis G Virus is a Flavivirus */fla' vi' vi'rus/*.

Hepatitis G is transmitted via contaminated blood transfusions and infected needle sticks.

There is no current treatment documented for Hepatitis G.

Human T-Cell Luekemia/Lymphoma Virus (HTLV-1)

The Human T-Cell (HTLV-1) Virus causes Adult T-Cell Leukemia/Lymphoma, which proves to be rapidly fatal. This virus is also associated with tropical Spastic Paresis and Multiple Sclerosis.

The Human T-Cell (HTLV-1) Virus is a double stranded positive sense RNA Retroviridae */ret' ro vir' ide/* Virus.

The Human T-Cell (HTLV-1) Virus develops by infecting and transforming normal cells into malignant cells that lose contact inhibition and pile up in vitro.

There is no current treatment or prevention for the Human T-Cell (HTLV-1) Virus.

Human T-Cell Luekemia/Lymphoma Virus (HTLV-2)

The Human T-Cell (HTLV-2) Virus causes T-Hairy Cell Leukemia.

The Human T-Cell (HTLV-2) Virus is a double stranded positive sense RNA Retroviridae */ret' ro vir' ide/* Virus.

The Human T-Cell (HTLV-2) Virus develops by infecting and transforming normal cells into malignant cells that loose contact inhibition and pile up in vitro.

There is no current treatment or prevention for the Human T-Cell (HTLV-1) Virus.

Human Immunodeficiency Virus (HIV Є" 1)

The Human Immunodeficiency Virus (HIV-1) causes AIDS.

The Human Immunodeficiency Virus (HIV-1) Virus is a double stranded positive sense RNA Retroviridae */ret' ro vir' ide/* Virus.

The Human Immunodeficiency Virus (HIV-1) develops by binding to the T-Cells and the viral envelope fuses with the infected host cell, allowing capsid entry. The HIV Virus is transmitted in two ways: (1) 90% of cases are among homosexuals and IV drug users, with more males infected than females and (2) in Africa, HIV is spread heterosexually with equal numbers of males and females infected.

Transmission of HIV occurs, most commonly, via sexual activity. It can also occur via blood transfusions, IV needle sharing, infected mother to placenta, accidental contaminated needle stick among health care workers, and a very slight risk of contamination via contact of broken skin with contaminated body fluids.

Current treatment for (HIV-1) is Azidothymidine, Dideoxyinosine, and Dideoxycytidine.

Human Immunodeficiency Virus (HIV- 2)

The Human Immunodeficiency Virus (HIV-2) is the cause of AIDS in Western Africa.

The Human Immunodeficiency Virus (HIV-2) Virus is a double stranded positive sense RNA Retroviridae */ret' ro vir' ide/* Virus.

The Human Immunodeficiency Virus (HIV-2) develops by binding to the T-Cells and the viral envelope fuses with the infected host cell, allowing capsid entry.

There is no current treatment or prevention for HIV-2.

Herpes Simplex Virus-1 (HSV-1)

The Herpes Simplex Virus-1 (HSV-1) causes Gingivostomatitis. This causes painful blisters on the lips and mouth area. Fever and viral type symptoms often accompany these ulcers. Complications include Herpetic Keratitis of the eye and Encephalitis.

The Herpes Simplex Virus-1 (HSV-1) is a double-stranded linear DNA Herpesviridae */hur' pez' vir' ide/* Virus.

The Herpes Simplex Virus-1 (HSV-1) is transmitted by direct contact with the mucous membranes and sexual transmission.

The Herpes Simplex Virus-1 (HSV-1) is treated with Acyclovir, Trifluridine (topical) for corneal infection and Famciclovir.

Herpes Simplex Virus 2 (HSV-2)

The Herpes Simplex Virus 2 (HSV-2) causes Genital Herpes and Neonatal Herpes. Side effects include fever and viral symptoms.

The Herpes Simplex Virus 2 (HSV-2) is a double stranded linear DNA Herpesviridae */hur' pez' vir' ide/* Virus.

The Herpes Simplex Virus 2 (HSV-2) is transmitted sexually and via direct contact of the infected individuals mucous membranes.

The Herpes Simplex Virus 2 (HSV-2) is treated with Acyclovir and can be prevented by using condoms.

Varicella-Zoster Virus

The Varicella-Zoster */ver' isel' a zos' ter/* Virus causes chickenpox and shingles.

The Varicella- Zoster Virus is a double stranded DNA Herpesviridae */hur' pez vir' ide/* Virus.

The Varicella-Zoster /ver' isel' a zos' ter/ Virus is transmitted via respiratory secretions and direct contact with the ruptured blisters. This virus is extremely contagious.

The Varicella-Zoster Virus is treated with Acyclovir and Zoster Immune Globin. It is prevented with a new vaccine.

Cytomegalovirus

The Cytomegalovirus /si' tomeg' alovi' rus/ causes asympotomatic infections, infection of the fetus by toxoplasmosis and Cytomegalovirus /si' tomeg' alovi' ru/ Mononucleosis.

The Cytomegalovirus /si' tomeg' alovi' rus/ is a double stranded linear DNA Herpesviridae /hur' pez vir' ide/ Virus.

The Cytomegalovirus /ssi' tomeg' alovi' rus/ is transmitted via infected milk, saliva, urine, tears and sexually.

The Cytomegalovirus /si' tomeg' alovi' rus/ is treated with Foscarnet, Ganciclovir, Cidofovir, and Fomivirsen.

Epstein-Barr Virus (EBV)

The Epstein-Barr /ep' stin' bar'/ Virus causes infectious Mononucleosis with side effects of fever, sore throat, severe lethargy and enlarged lymph nodes and spleen.

The Epstein-Barr /ep' stin' bar'/ Virus is a double stranded linear DNA Herpesviridae /hur' pez vir' ide/ Virus.

The Epstein-Barr /ep' stin' bar'/ Virus is transmitted via intimate contact.

The Epstein-Barr /ep' stin' bar'/ Virus is treated with supportive care.

Human Herpesvirus 6 (HHV-6)

The Human Herpesvirus /hur' pez vi' rus/ causes Roseola. Side effects include high fever lasting for several days followed by a one to two day rash.

The Human Herpesvirus /hur' pez vi' rus/ 6 (HHV-6) is a double stranded DNA Herpesviridae /hur' pez vir' ide/ Virus.

The Human Herpesvirus /hur' pez vi' rus/ 6 (HHV-6) is transmitted via infected saliva.

There is no treatment for the Human Herpesvirus /hur' pez vi' rus/ 6.

HHV-8 Virus

The HHV 8 Virus appears to be the cause of Kaposi's Sarcona.

The HHV-8 Virus is a double stranded DNA Herpesviridae /hur' pez vir' ide/ Virus.

The HHV-8 Virus is transmitted sexually, particularly in homosexual males.

The HHV-8 has no current treatment.

POXviridae Virus

The POXviridae /poks' vir' ide/ Virus causes Small Pox and Molluscum Contagiosum.

The POXviridae /*poks' vir' ide*/ Virus is a complex coat double stranded linear DNA Virus. This is the only virus capable of replicating in cytoplasm.

The POXviridae /*poks' vir' ide*/ Virus has been eradicated from the Earth. At one time, it was highly contagious and spread via the respiratory tract.

A vaccine of an Avirulent Pox Virus, which induces immunity to the virulent pox virus, prevents the POXviridae /*poks' vir' ide*/ Virus.

PAPOVAvirdae Virus

The PAPOVAvirdae /*pap' ova' vir' ide*/ Virus causes the Human Papilloma Virus (HPV) which causes warts. This includes common warts, genital warts, laryngeal warts, and cervical cancer.

The PAPOVAVirdae /*pap' ova' vir' ide*/ Virus is a naked Icosohedral /*i ko' so' he' dral*/ Double Stranded DNA Papovaviridae /*pap' ova' vir' ide*/ Virus.

The PAPOVAVirdae /*pap' ova' vir' ide*/ Virus is omnipresent, but many people do not develop warts for unknown reasons.

The PAPOVAVirdae /*pap' ova' vir' ide*/ Virus is treated with removal of the warts by: freezing them, surgically removing them, laser ablation, and Padophyllin (for genital warts). It is important to note that most warts will resolve spontaneously in 1-2 years, but relapses are common.

ADENOviridae Virus

The ADENOViridae /ad' eno' vir' ide/ Virus causes childhood respiratory infections with the side effects of Rhinitis, sore throat, fever and Conjunctivitis.

The ADENOViridae /ad' eno' vir' ide/ Virus is a naked Icosohedral /i ko' so' he' dral/ Double Stranded Linear DNA Virus.

Coughing and sneezing among children spreads the ADENOViridae /ad' eno' vir' ide/ Virus.

The ADENOViridae /ad' eno' vir' ide/ Virus is self-limited and no treatment is necessary.

PARVOviridae Virus

The PARVOvirdae /par' vo' vir' ide/ Virus causes Fifth Disease. Complications include a fever and slight rash.

The PARVOvirdae /par' vo' vir' ide/ Virus is a naked Icosohedral /i ko' so' he' dral/ Single Stranded Linear DNA Virus.

The PARVOvirdae /par' vo' vir' ide/ Virus is self-limited and no treatment is necessary.

Alpha Virus

The Alpha Virus causes the Encephalitis Viruses which includes symptoms of headaches, fever, altered level of consciousness and focal neurologic deficits.

The Alpha Virus is a positive single stranded RNA TOGAvirdae /to' ga' vir' ide/ Virus.

The Alpha Virus is transmitted via infected mosquitoes.

The Alpha Virus is prevented with mosquito control mechanisms.

Rubivirus

Rubivirus /roo' bevi' rus/ causes the 3 day measles and German measles. Side effects include congenital defects, if an expectant mother is exposed during the first trimester of pregnancy.

The Rubivirus /roo' bevi' rus/ is a positive single stranded RNA TOGAvirdae /to' ga' vir' ide/ Virus.

Respiratory secretions spread the Rubivirus /roo' bevi' rus/.

The Rubivirus /roo' bevi' rus/ is prevented with the MMR (Measles, Mumps, Rubella) Vaccine.

Yellow Fever Virus

The Yellow Fever Virus causes Hepatitis with Jaundice. Symptoms include fever and a backache.

The Yellow Fever Virus is a positive single stranded RNA FLAVviridae /fla' v' - vir' ide/ Virus.

The Yellow Fever Virus is spread via infected mosquitoes.

The Yellow Fever Virus is prevented with mosquito control mechanisms.

Dengue Virus

The Dengue /deng' ge/ Virus causes Dengue /deng' ge/ Fever, also known as Break Bone Fever. This is a painful fever accompanied by headache, muscle aches, joint aches and a back ache.

The Dengue /deng' ge/ Virus is a positive single stranded RNA FLAVviridae /fla' v' - vir' ide/ Virus.

The Dengue /deng' ge/ Virus is spread via infected mosquitoes.

The Dengue /deng' ge/ Virus is prevented with mosquito control.

St. Louis Encephalitis Virus

The St. Louis Encephalitis Virus causes Encephalitis accompanied by fever.

The St. Louis Encephalitis Virus is a positive single stranded RNA FLAVviridae /fla' v' vir' ide/ Virus.

The St. Louis Encephalitis Virus is spread via infected mosquitoes.

The St. Louis Encephalitis Virus is prevented with mosquito control mechanisms.

Japanese Encephalitis Virus

The Japanese Encephalitis Virus causes Encephalitis accompanied by fever.

The Japanese Encephalitis Virus is a positive single stranded RNA FLAVviridae /fla' v' - vir' ide/ Virus.

The Japanese Encephalitis Virus is spread via infected mosquitoes.

The Japanese Encephalitis Virus is prevented with mosquito control mechanisms.

Hepatitis C Virus

The Hepatitis C Virus causes Hepatitis C.

The Hepatitis C Virus is a positive single stranded RNA FLAVviridae /fla' v' - vir' ide/ Virus.

The Hepatitis C Virus is spread via infected mosquitoes.

The Hepatitis C Virus is prevented with mosquito control mechanisms.

California Encephalitis Virus

The California Encephalitis Virus causes fever and Encephalitis.

The California Encephalitis Virus is a negative single stranded RNA BUNYAviridae /bun' ya' vir' ide/ Virus.

The California Encephalitis Virus is spread via infected mosquitoes.

The California Encephalitis Virus is prevented with mosquito control mechanisms.

Rift Valley Fever Virus

The Rift Valley Fever Virus causes fever and Encephalitis.

The Rift Valley Fever Virus is a negative single stranded RNA BUNYAviridae /*bun' ya' vir' ide*/ Virus.

The Rift Valley Fever Virus is spread via infected mosquitoes.

The Rift Valley Fever Virus is prevented with mosquito control mechanisms.

Sandfly Fever Virus

The Sandfly Fever Virus causes fever and Encephalitis.

The Sandfly Fever Virus is a negative single stranded RNA BUNYAviridae /*bun' ya' vir' ide*/ Virus.

The Sandfly Fever Virus is spread via infected mosquitoes.

The Sandfly Fever Virus is prevented with mosquito control mechanisms.

Hanaivirus

The Hantavirus causes Hemorrhagic Fever with Renal Syndrome in Europe and Asia and Hantavirus Pulmonary Syndrome in New Mexico, Arizona, Colorado and Utah. Symptoms include fever, muscle aches, cough, nausea, vomiting and pulmonary edema which leads to respiratory failure.

The Hantavirus is a negative single stranded RNA BUNYAviridae *bun' ya' vir' ide*/ Virus.

Many believe the Hantavirus spread by rodents, but the actual mechanism is unknown.

The Hantavirus is currently treated in investigations by Ribavirin.

Poliovirus

The Polio Virus causes mild Febrile illness in infants, Aseptic Meningitis, and Paralytic Poliomyelitis.

The Polio Virus is a positive single stranded RNA ENTEROviridae */en' tiro' vir' ide/* virus.

The Polio Virus is transmitted fecally and orally and also by respiratory secretions of infected individuals.

Current prevention for the Polio Virus is the Salk Vaccine and the Oral Polio Vaccine.

Coxsackie A Virus

The Coxsackie */koksak' e/* A Virus causes the common cold, rashes and Viral Meningitis. It is also the cause of the Hand Foot and Mouth Disease in children and Herpangina.

The Coxsackie */koksak' e/* A Virus is a positive single stranded RNA ENTEROviridae */en' tiro vir' ide/* virus.

The Coxsackie */koksak' e/* A Virus is spread via direct contact.

The Coxsackie */koksak' e/* A Virus is treated with supportive care. The Coxsackie A Virus can be prevented with proper hand washing practices.

Coxsackie B Virus

The Coxsackie /koksak' e/ B Virus causes Viral Meningitis, Arthymia, Cardiomyopathy and hear failure.

The Coxsackie /koksak' e/ B Virus is a positive single stranded RNA ENTEROviridae /en' tiro vir' ide/ Virus.

The Coxsackie /koksak' e/ B Virus is spread via direct contact.

The Coxsackie /koksak' e/ B Virus is treated with supportive care and can be prevented with proper hand washing practices.

ECHOvirus

The ECHOvirus /ek' ovi' rus/ causes the common cold, rashes, Viral Meningitis and Pericarditis.

The Echovirus //ek' ovi' rus/ is a positive single stranded RNA ENTEROviridae /en' tiro vir' ide/ Virus.

The Echovirus //ek' ovi' rus/ is spread via direct contact.

The Echovirus //ek' ovi' rus/ is treated with supportive care and can be prevented with proper hand washing practices.

Hepatitis A Virus

The Hepatitis A Virus causes infectious Hepatitis, fever, Jaundice and elevated liver enzymes.

The Hepatitis A Virus is a positive single stranded RNA ENTEROviridae /en' tiro vir' ide/ Virus.

The Hepatitis A Virus is transmitted via the feces of the

infected person or orally.

The Hepatitis A Virus is treated with supportive care. It can be prevented with the new HAV Vaccine.

Rhinovirus

There are 113 stereotypes of the Rhinovirus. The Rhinovirus is responsible for the common cold.

The Rhinovirus is a positive single stranded Rhinoviridae /rino' vir' ide/ virus.

The Rhinovirus is spread via direct contact.

The Rhinovirus is treated with supportive care.

Norwalk Virus

The Norwalk Virus causes Viral Gastroenteritis. Symptoms include diarrhea, fever, abdominal pain, and vomiting. This can be fatal for infants due to the loss of fluids and electrolytes.

The Norwalk Virus is a positive single stranded RNA Caliciviridae /kalis' i vir' ide/ Virus.

The Norwalk Virus is transmitted via the feces of the infected person and orally.

The Norwalk Virus is treated with intravenous fluids.

Calciviruses

The Calciviruses /kalis' i vir' ide/ cause viral Gastroenteritis and possibly Hepatitis E.

The Calciviruses /kalis' i vir' ide/ are a positive single stranded RNA Caliciviridae /kalis' i vir' ide/ Virus.

The Calciviruses /kalis' i vir' ide/ are transmitted via the feces of the infected person and orally.

The Calciviruses /kalis' i vir' ide/ are treated with intravenous fluids.

Rotavirus

The Rotavirus /ro' tovi' rus/ causes Gastroenteritis with severe dehydration (especially in infants), fever, abdominal pain, vomiting and diarrhea.

The Rotavirus /ro' tovi' rus/ is a double stranded RNA Reoviridae /re' o vir' ide/ Virus.

The Rotavirus /ro' tovi' rus/ is transmitted via the feces of the infected person and orally.

The Rotavirus /ro' tovi' rus/ is treated with intravenous fluids. There is a new oral Rotavirus Vaccine that appears to be safe for infants.

Coronaviridae Virus

The Coronaviridae /kor' ona vir' ide/ Virus is the cause of the common upper respiratory infection.

The Coronaviridae /kor' ona vir' ide/ Virus is a positive single stranded RNA Coronaviridae /kor' ona vir' ide/ Virus.

The Coronaviridae /kor' ona vir' ide/ Virus is transmitted via mucous secretions and hand to hand contact.

The Coronaviridae /kor' ona vir' ide/ Virus is treated with supportive care.

Rabies Virus

The Rabies Virus causes rabies. Symptoms include fever, headache, sore throat and heightened sensitivity around the wound site. In severe cases, it can also cause acute Encephalitis leading to confusion and seizures.

The Rabies Virus is a negative single stranded RNA Rhabdoviridae /rab' do vir' ide/ Virus.

The Rabies Virus is transmitted via an infected animal bite.

The Rabies Virus is treated by passive immunization with the Rabies Immune Globin and with active immunization of killed Rabies Virus Vaccine. The virus is prevented by vaccination of animals.

Marburg Virus

The Marburg Virus causes Acute Viral Hemorrhagic Fever with a high mortality rate.

The Marburg Virus is a negative single stranded RNA Filoviridae /fi' lo vir' ide/ Virus.

The Marburg Virus is transmitted via contact with infected body fluids.

The Marburg Virus is treated with supportive therapy.

Ebola Virus

The Ebola Virus causes fever, headache, myalgia, abdominal pain, diarrhea, Pharyngitis, hiccups, cough and somnolence can develop. This eventually results in death from organ failure.

The Ebola Virus is a negative single stranded RNA Filoviridae */fi' lo vir' ide/* Virus.

The Ebola Virus is transmitted via contact with infected body fluids.

The Ebola Virus is treated with supportive therapy.

Lymphocytic Choriomeningitis Virus

The Lymphocytic */lim' fosit' ik/* Choriomeningitis Virus causes Lymphocytic */lim' fosit' ik/*Choriomeningitis with influenza symptoms.

The Lymphocytic */lim' fosit' ik/* Choriomeningitis Virus is a negative single stranded RNA Arenaviridae */er' ina vir' ide/* Virus.

The Lymphocytic */lim' fosit' ik/* Choriomeningitis Virus is spread via rodent urine.

The Lymphocytic /lim' fosit' ik/ Choriomeningitis Virus is treated with supportive care.

Lassa Virus

The Lassa Virus causes Lassa Fever with symptoms of fever, sore throat, abdominal pain, and vomiting. This can be fatal 50% of the time.

The Lassa Virus is a negative single stranded RNA Arenaviridae /er' ina vir' ide/ Virus.

The Lassa Virus is spread via rodent urine.

The Lassa Virus is treated with Ribavirin /ri' bavir' in/.

Bacteria

A numerous group of microscopic single celled organisms are called bacteria. A variety of these species cause infectious diseases.

Streptococcus Pyogenes Bacteria

The Streptococcus /strep' tokok' us/ Pyogenes /pi' ojens/ Bacteria causes Pharyngitis or Strep Throat, skin infections (including Folliculitis, Cellulitis and Impetigo), Scarlet Fever and Toxic Shock Syndrome. It can also cause the Flesh Eating Streptococcus. Severe cases of Strep Throat can result in Rheumatic Fever.

The Streptococcus /strep' tokok' us/ Pyogenes /pi' ojens/ Bacteria is a Gram-Positive Cocci Lancefield Group A Bacteria.

The Streptococcus /strep' tokok' us/ Pyogenes /pi' ojens/ Bacteria expresses the following virulence factors; M-protein (70 types), Lipoteichoic Acid, Streptokinase, Hyaluronidase, DNAase, and Antic-C5a peptidase.

Penicillin G, Penicillin V, and Erthromycin are all used to treat Streptococcus /strep' tokok' us/ Pyogenes /pi' ojens/. Clindamycin is added for invasive Streptococcus /strep' tokok' us/ Pyogenes /pi' ojens/ infections. If a patient develops Rheumatic Fever, they are placed on continuous prophylactic Antibiotics.

Streptococcus Agalactiae Bacteria

The Streptococcus /strep' tokok' us/ Agalactiae /a' galak' ti/ Bacteria causes Neonatal Meningitis, Pneumonia, and Sepsis.

The Streptococcus /strep' tokok' us/ Agalactiae /a' galak' ti/ Bacteria is a Catalase-Negative Lancefield Group B Cocci Bacteria.

The Streptococcus /strep' tokok' us/ Agalactiae /a' galak' ti/ Bacteria is less virulent and expresses few virulence factors.

Penicillin G is used to treat Streptococcus /strep' tokok' us/ Agalactiae /a' galak' ti/.

Enterococcus Faecalis Bacteria

The Enterococcus /en' tero kokus/ Faecalis /fak' alis/ Bacteria causes Subacute Bacterial Endocarditis, binary tract infections and urinary tract infections.

TheEnterococcus /en' tero kokus/ Faecalis /fak' alis/ Bacteria is a Catalase-Negative Lancefield Group D Enterococcus /en' tero kokus/ Bacteria.

The Enterococcus /en' tero kokus/ Faecalis /fak' alis /Bacteria is less virulent and expresses few virulence factors.

Ampicillan combined with an aminoglycoside is used to treat theEnterococcus /en' tero kokus/ Faecalis /fak' alis/ Bacteria. This bacteria is resistant to Penicillin G.

Enterococcus Faecium Bacteria

The Enterococcus /en' tero kokus/ Faecium /fak' ium/ Bacteria causes Subacute Bacterial Endocarditis, binary tract infections and urinary tract infections.

 The Enterococcus /en' tero kokus/ Faecium /fak' ium/ Bacteria is a Catalase-Negative Lancefield Group D Enterococcus /en' tero kokus/ Bacteria.

The Enterococcus /en' tero kokus/ Faecium /fak' ium/ Bacteria is less virulent and expresses few virulence factors.

Ampicillan combined with an Aminoglycoside is used to treat the Enterococcus //en' tero kokus/ Faecium /fak' ium/ Bacteria. This bacteria is resistant to Penicillin G.

Streptococcus Bovis Bacteria

The Streptococcus /strep' to kok' us/ Bovis /bo' vis/ Bacteria causes Subacute Bacterial Endocarditis, binary tract infections and urinary tract infections.

The Streptococcus /strep' to kok' us/ Bovis /bo' vis/ Bacteria is a Catalase-Negative Lancefield Group D Non-Enterococci /en' tero koki/ Bacteria.

The Streptococcus /strep' to kok' us/ Bovis /bo' vis/ Bacteria is less virulent and expresses few virulence factors.

Ampicillan combined with an Aminoglycoside is used to treat the Streptococcus /strep' to kok' us/ Bovis /bo' vis/ Bacteria. This bacteria is resistant to Penicillin G.

Streptococcus Equinus Bacteria

The Streptococcus /strep' to kok' us/ Equinus /ekwi' nus/ Bacteria causes Subacute Bacterial Endocarditis, binary tract infections and urinary tract infections.

The Streptococcus /strep' to kok' us/ Equinus /ekwi' nus/ Bacteria is a Catalase-Negative Lancefield Group D Non-Enterococci Bacteria.

The Streptococcus /strep' to kok' us/ Equinus /ekwi' nus/ Bacteria is less virulent and expresses few virulence factors.

Ampicillan combined with an aminoglycoside is used to treat the Streptococcus /strep' to kok' us/ Equinus /ekwi' nus/ Bacteria. This bacteria is resistant to Penicillin G.

Viridans Streptococci Bacteria

The Viridans /vir' i dans/ Streptococci /strep' tokok' i/ Bacteria causes Subacute Bacterial Endocarditis, dental cavities and brain and liver abscesses.

The Viridans /vir' i dans/ Streptococci /strep' tokok' i/ Bacteria is a Catalase /kat' alas/ Negative Cocci Bacteria.

The Viridans /vir' i dans/ Streptococci /strep' tokok' i/ Bacteria expresses the following potential virulence factors; extracellular dextran that helps them bond to heart valves.

Penicillin G is used to treat Viridans /vir' i dans/ Streptococci /strep' tokok' i/ Bacteria.

Streptococcus Pneumonia (Pneumococci) Bacteria

The Streptococcus /strep' tokok' us/ Pneumonia /noomo' ne a/ (Pneumococci) /noomo' koki/ Bacteria causes Pneumonia, Meningitis, Sepsis and Otitis Media in children.

The Streptococcus /strep' tokok' us/ Pneumonia /noomo' ne a/ (Pneumococci) /noomo' koki/ Bacteria is a Catalase-Negative Cocci Bacteria.

The Streptococcus /strep' tokok' is/ Pneumonia /noomo' ne a/ (Pneumococci) /noomo' koki/ Bacteria has 83 serotypes of capsule as a potential virulence factor.

Pencillin G, Erthyromycin, and Ceftriaxone are used to treat the Streptococcus /strep' tokok' us/ Pneumonia /noomo' ne a/ (Pneumococci) /noomo' koki/ Bacteria. A vaccine has been developed for the 23 most common capsular antigens and is being used for prevention.

Staphylococcus Aeurus Bacteria

The Staphylococcus /staf' ilokok' us/ Aerus /or' e us/ Bacteria causes food poisoning with the rapid onset of vomiting and diarrhea and vomiting. It can also cause Toxic Shock Syndrome, Pneumonia, Meningitis, Osteomyelitis, Acute Bacterial Endocarditis and Septic Arthritis.

The Staphylococcus /staf' ilokok' us/ Aerus /or' e us/ Bacteria is a Catalase positive Cocci Bacteria.

The Staphylococcus /staf' ilokok' us/ Aerus /or' e us/ Bacteria expresses the following virulence factors; Protein A binds IgG which prevents opsonization and phagocytosis, Coagulase allows fibrin formation around the organism, Hemolysins, Leukocidins, and Penicillinase. The tissue destroying proteins react in the following manner: the Hyaluronidase breaks down the connective tissue, the Staphylokinase Lyses formed clots, and Lipase.

Penicillinase, Vancomycin, and Clindamycin are used to treat the Staphylococcus /staf' ilokok' us/ Aerus /or' e us/ Bacteria.

Staphylococcus Epidermidis Bacteria

The Staphylococcus /staf' ilokok' us/ Epidermidis /ep' idurmi' tis/ Bacteria causes Nosocomial Infections and is a frequent contaminant in blood cultures.

The Staphylococcus /staf' ilokok' us/ Epidermidis /ep' idurmi' tis/ Bacteria is a Catalase-Positive Cocci Bacteria.

Staphylococcus staf' ilokok' us/ Epidermidis /ep' idurmi' tis/ Bacteria has the following virulence factors; a Polysaccharide Capsule that adheres to a variety of prosthetic devices and is highly resistant to antibiotics.

Vancomycin is used to treat Staphylococcus /staf' ilokok' us/ Epidermidis /ep' idurmi' tis/ Bacteria.

Staphylococcus Saprophyticus Bacteria

The Staphylococcus /staf' ilokok' us/ Saprophyticus /sap' rofit kus/ Bacteria causes urinary tract infections in sexually active women.

The Staphylococcus /staf' ilokok' us/ Saprophyticus /sap' rofit kus/ Bacteria is a Catalase-Positive Cocci Bacteria.

The Staphylococcus /*staf' ilokok' us*/ Saprophyticus /*sap' rofit kus*/ Bacteria is less virulent and expresses few virulence factors.

The Staphylococcus /*staf' ilokok' us*/ Saprophyticus /*sap' rofit kus*/ Bacteria is treated with Penicillin.

Bacillus Anthracis Bacteria

The Bacillus /*ba' sil' us*/ Anthracis /*an' thrak sis*/ Bacteria causes painless black vesicles that can be fatal if left untreated. Additionally, it causes Woolsorter's Disease. Symptoms include abdominal pain, vomiting and bloody diarrhea.

The Bacillus /*ba' sil' us*/ Anthracis /*an' thrak sis*/ Bacteria is a Herbavore Zoonotic Bacillus Gram Positive Spore-Forming Rod Bacteria. It is Aerobic, but because it can grow without oxygen, it is classified as a Facultative Anaerobe.

The Bacillus /*ba' sil' us*/ Anthracis /*an' thrak sis*/ Bacteria expresses the following virulence factors; unique protein capsule of polymer gamma-D-Glumatic Acid anti-phagocytic, non-motile, and the virulence depends on acquiring 2 plasmids. One carries the gene for the protein capsule and the other carries the gene for the exotoxin.

The Bacillus /*ba' sil' us*/ Anthracis /*an' thrak sis*/ Bacteria is transmitted through endospores via cutaneous, inhalation or ingestion.

The Bacillus /*ba' sil' us*/ Anthracis /*an' thrak sis*/ Bacteria is treated with Penicillin G and Erthromycin. A vaccine of protective antigen is available for high risk individuals.

Bacillus Cereus Bacteria

The Bacillus /*basil' us*/ Cereus /*ser' e us*/ Bacteria causes food poisoning with symptoms of diarrhea, nausea and vomiting.

The Bacillus /*basil' us*/ Cereus /*ser' e us*/ Bacteria is an Aerobic Bacillus Gram-Positive Spore-Forming Rod Bacteria. It is transmitted through endospores.

The Bacillus /*basil' us*/ Cereus /*ser' e us*/Bacteria has a non-capsule motile virulence factor.

The Bacillus /*basil' us*/ Cereus /*ser' e us*/ Bacteria is treated with Vancomycin and Clindamycin. It is resistant to Beta Lactam Antibiotics.

Clostridium Botulinum Bacteria

The Clostridium /*klostrid' e um*/ Botulinum /*boch' ulin um*/ Bacteria causes Botulism in food with symptoms of cranial nerve palsies, muscle weakness, and respiratory paralysis.

The Clostridium /*klostrid' e um*/ Botulinum /*boch' ulin um*/ Bacteria is an Anaerobic Gram-Positive Spore-Forming Rod Bacteria.

The Clostridium /*klostrid' e um*/ Botulinum /*boch' ulin um*/ Bacteria has a motile flagella virulence factor.

The Clostridium /*klostrid' e um*/ Botulinum /*boch' ulin um*/ Bacteria is transmitted via heat resistant endospores.

The Clostridium /klostrid' e um/ Botulinum /boch' ulin um/ Bacteria is treated with Antitoxin, Penicillin, Hyperbaric Oxygen and supportive therapy.

Clostridium Tetani Bacteria

The Clostridium /klostrid' e um/ Tetani /tet' ane/ Bacteria causes Tetnus. Symptoms include muscle spasms, lockjaw, Risus Sardonicus, and respiratory muscle paralysis.

The Clostridium /klostrid' e um/ Tetani /tet' ane/ Bacteria is an Anaerobic Gram-Positive Spore-Forming Rod Bacteria.

The Clostridium /klostrid' e um/ Tetani /tet' ane/ Bacteria is transmitted via endospores that enter the wound.

The Clostridium /klostrid' e um/ Tetani /tet' ane/ Bacteria has a motile flagella virulence factor.

The Clostridium /klostrid' e um/ Tetani /tet' ane/ Bacteria is treated with Penicillin or Metronidazole. The DPT Vaccine prevents it.

Clostridium Perfringens Bacteria

The Clostridium /klostrid' e um/ Perfringens /per' frin jens/ Bacteria causes Gasseous Gangrene, Cellulitis and Clostridial Myonecrosis.

The Clostridium /klostrid' e um/ Perfringens /per' frin jens/ Bacteria is an Anaerobic Gram-Positive Spore-Forming Rod Bacteria.

The Clostridium /klostrid' e um/ Perfringens /per' frin jens/ Bacteria is transmitted via endospores.

The Clostridium /klostrid' e um/ Perfringens /per' frin jens/ Bacteria has a non-motile virulence factor.

The Clostridium /klostrid' e um/ Perfringens /per' frin jens/ Bacteria is treated with surgery, which may require amputation, Penicillin and Clindamycin, and Hyperbaric Oxygen.

Clostridium Difficile Bacteria

The Clostridium /klostrid' e um/ Difficile /difis' ile/ Bacteria causes Pseudomembranous.

The Clostridium /klostrid' e um/ Difficile /difis' ile/ Bacteria is an Anaerobic Gram-Positive Spore-Forming Rod Bacteria.

The Clostridium /klostrid' e um/ Difficile /difis' ile/ Bacteria is transmitted fecally or orally via ingestion of spores.

The Clostridium /klostrid' e um/ Difficile /difis' ile/ Bacteria has a motile flagella virulence factor.

The Clostridium /klostrid' e um/ Difficile /difis' ile/ Bacteria is treated with Metronidazole and oral Vancomycin.

Corynebacterium Diphtheriae Bacteria

The Corynebacterium /kor' ine' baktir' e um/ Diphtheriae /difthir' ei/ Bacteria causes Diptheria. Initial symptoms include a mild sore throat with fever. Followed by pseudomembrane that forms on the Pharynx, Myocarditis, and neural involvement.

The Corynebacterium /kor' ine' baktir' e um/ Diphtheriae /difthir' ei/ Bacteria is a Facultative Anaerobe Catalase Gram Positive Non-Spore Forming Rod.

The Corynebacterium /kor' ine' baktir' e um/ Diphtheriae /difthir' ei/ Bacteria is transmitted via respiratory droplets from a carrier.

The Corynebacterium /kor' ine' baktir' e um/ Diphtheriae /difthir' ei/ Bacteria virulence factors include a Pseudomembrane forming in the pharynx, which serves as the focal point for where the toxin is created.

The Corynebacterium /kor' ine' baktir' e um/ Diphtheriae /difthir' ei/ Bacteria is treated with antitoxin and Penicillin or Erythromycin. It is prevented with the DPT Vaccine.

Listeria Monocytogenes Bacteria

The Listeria/lister' ea/ Monocytogenes /mon' ositoj' inez/ Bacteria causes Neonatal Meningitis and Septicemia.

The Listeria/lister' ea/ Monocytogenes /mon' ositoj' inez/ Bacteria is Facultative Anaerobe Catalase Gram Positive Non Spore Forming Rod.

The Listeria/lister' ea/ Monocytogenes /mon' ositoj' inez/ Bacteria is transmitted via ingestion of contaminated raw milk or cheese from infected cows and vaginally during birth.

The Listeria/lister' ea/ Monocytogenes /mon' ositoj' inez/ Bacteria expresses the following virulence factors; motile via flagella and Hemolysin.

The Listeria/*lister' ea*/ Monocytogenes /*mon' ositoj' inez*/ Bacteria is treated with Ampicillin and Trimethoprim/Sulfamethoxazole.

Neisseria Meningococcus Bacteria

The Neisseria /*niser' ea*/ Meningococcus /*mining' gokok' us*/ Bacteria causes asymptomatic carriage in the Nasopharynx, Meningitis, and septicemia.

The Neisseria /*niser' ea*/ Meningococcus /*mining' gokok' us*/ Bacteria is a Gram-Negative Diplococci Faculatative Anaerobe Neisseria Bacteria.

The Neisseria /*niser' ea*/ Meningococcus /*mining' gokok' us*/ Bacteria is spread by respiratory transmission from infected humans.

The Neisseria /*niser' ea*/ Meningococcus /*mining' gokok' us*/ Bacteria expresses the following virulence factors; capsule with nine serotypes, IgA1 protease, can extract iron from transferrin, and a pill for adherence.

The Neisseria /*niser' ea*/ Meningococcus /*mining' gokok' us*/ Bacteria is treated with Penicillin, Ceftriaxone and Rifampin. There is also a vaccine against capsular antigens A, C, Y and W-135, but not B.

Neisseria Gonorrhea Bacteria

The Neisseria /*niser' ea*/ Gonorrhea /gon' ore' a/ Bacteria causes Urethritis in men and Cervical Gonorrhea in women, which can progress, to PID. It also causes Gonococcal Bacteremia, Septic Arthritis and Neonates in both men and women.

The Neisseria /niser' ea/ Gonorrhea /gon' rre'a/ Bacteria is a Gram Negative Diplococci Facultative-Anaerobe Neisseria /niser' ea/ Bacteria.

The Neisseria /niser' ea/ Gonorrhea /gon' rre'a/ Bacteria is spread via sexual transmission.

The Neisseria /niser' ea/ Gonorrhea /gon' rre'a/ Bacteria expresses the following virulence factors; the pill, IgA1 protease, and outer membrane proteins.

The Neisseria /niser' ea/ Gonorrhea /gon' rre'a/ Bacteria is treated with third generation Cephalosporin such as Ceftriaxone. To prevent Opthaimia Neonatorum, Erythromycin eye drops are given immediately following birth.

Branhamella Catarrhalis Bacteria

The Branhamella /bran' ham ella/ Catarrhalis /kat' ur alis/ Bacteria causes Ottis Media in children and other types of respiratory infections.

The Branhamella /bran' ham ella/ Catarrhalis /kat' ur alis/ Bacteria is a Gram Negative Diplococci Facultative-Anaerobe Neisseria Bacteria.

The Branhamella /bran' ham ella/ Catarrhalis /kat' ur alis/ Bacteria is part of the normal respiratory flora.

The Branhamella /bran' ham ella/ Catarrhalis /kat' ur alis/ Bacteria is treated with Zaithromycin or Clarithromycin, Amoxcillan with Clavulanate, Oral or second generation Cephalosporin, and Trimethroprim/Sulfamethoxazole.

Escherichia Coli Bacteria

The Escherichia /eshiri' ke a/ Coli /ko' li/ Bacteria causes newborn Meningitis, urinary tract infection, hospital acquired Sepsis, hospital acquired pneumonia and diarrhea.

The Escherichia /eshiri' ke a/ Coli /ko' li/ Bacteria is an Indole-Positive Catalase Facultative Anaerobic Enterobacteriaceae /en' tirobaktir' e a' si e/ Enteric Bacteria.

The Escherichia /eshiri' ke a/ Coli /ko' li/ Bacteria is transmitted in the following ways, fecal, oral migration up the urethra, colonization of catheters in hospitalized patients and aspiration of oral E. Coli.

The Virulence factors of The Escherichia /eshiri' ke a/ Coli /ko' li/ Bacteria include; a fimbriae colonization factor, siderophore, adhesins, capsule (K-Antigen), and flagella (H-Antigen).

The Escherichia /eshiri' ke a/ Coli /ko' li/ Bacteria is treated with Cephalosporins, Aminoglycosides, Trimethoprim & Sulfamethoxazole, and Fluoroquinolones.

Klebsiella Pneumoniae Bacteria

The Klebsiella /kleb' ze el' a/ Pneumoniae /noo mon' ye/ Bacteria causes Pneumonia, hospital acquired urinary tract infections and Sepsis.

The Klebsiella /kleb' ze el' a/ Pneumoniae /noo mon' ye/ Bacteria is an Indole-Negative Enteric Enterobacteriaceae /en' tirobaktir' e a' si e/ Bacteria.

The Klebsiella /kleb' ze el' a/ Pneumoniae /noo mon' ye/ Bacteria has a non-motile capsule virulence factor.

The Klebsiella /kleb' ze el' a/ Pneumoniae /noo mon' ye/ Bacteria is treated with third generation Cephalosporin and Ciprofloxacin.

Proteus Mirabilis Bacteria

The Proteus /pro' te us/ Mirabilis /mir' ab ilis/ Bacteria causes urinary tract infection and Sepsis.

The Proteus /pro' te us/ Mirabilis /mir' ab ilis/ Bacteria is an Indole-Negative Enterobacteriaceae /en' tirobaktir' e a' si e/ Enteric Bacteria.

The Proteus /pro' te us/ Mirabilis /mir' ab ilis/ Bacteria has a motile virulence factor.

The Proteus /pro' te us/ Mirabilis /mir' ab ilis/ Bacteria is treated with Ampicillin, Trimethoprim & Sulfamethoxazole.

Shigella Dysenteriae Bacteria

The Shigella /shigel' a/ Dysenteriae /dis' inter' e/ Bacteria causes bloody diarrhea with mucus and pus.

The Shigella /shigel' a/ Dysenteriae /dis' inter' e/ Bacteria is a Catalase Positive Enterobacteriaceae /en' tirobaktir' e a' si e/ Enteric Bacteria.

The Shigella /*shigel' a*/ Dysenteriae /*dis' inter' e*/ Bacteria has the following virulence factors; it invades submucosa of intestinal tract and it is non-motile.

The Shigella /*shigel' a*/ Dysenteriae /*dis' inter' e*/ Bacteria is transmitted orally and through infected feces.

Salmonella Typhi Bacteria

The Salmonella /*sal' monel' a*/ Typhi /*ti' fi*/ Bacteria causes Enteric Fever, chronic carrier state, Gastroenteritis, Sepsis, and Osteomyelitis.

The Salmonella /*sal' monel' a*/ Typhi /*ti' fi*/ Bacteria is a Catalase Positive Enterobacteriaceae /*en' tirobaktir' e a' si e*/ Enteric Bacteria.

The Salmonella /*sal' monel' a*/ Typhi /*ti' fi*/ Bacteria is transmitted via infected feces and orally.

The Salmonella /*sal' monel' a*/ Typhi /*ti' fi*/ Bacteria has the following virulence factors; motile, capsule and siderophore.

The Salmonella /*sal' monel' a*/ Typhi /*ti' fi*/ Bacteria is treated with Ciprofloxacin, Ceftriaxone, Trimethoprim & Sulfamethoxazzole and Azithromycin.

Non-Typhi Groups of Salmonella Bacteria

The Non-Typhi /*ti' fi*/ Groups of Salmonella /*sal' monel' a*/ Bacteria causes Enteric Fever, chronic carrier state, Gastroenteritis, Sepsis, and Osteomyelitis.

The Non-Typhi /ti' fi/ Groups of Salmonella /sal' monel' a/ Bacteria is a Catalase Positive Enterobacteriaceae /en' tirobaktir' e a' si e/ Enteric Bacteria.

The Non-Typhi /ti' fi/ Groups of Salmonella /sal' monel' a/ Bacteria is transmitted from infected pet turtles, chickens and uncooked eggs.

The Non-Typhi /ti' fi/ Groups of Salmonella /sal' monel' a/ Bacteria have the following virulence factors; it is motile, capsule and siderophore.

The Non-Typhi /ti' fi/ Groups of Salmonella /sal' monel' a/ Bacteria is treated with Ciprofloxacin, Ceftriaxone, Trimethoprim & Sulfamethoxazzole and Azithromycin.

Yersinia Enterocolitica Bacteria

The Yersinia /yersin' e a/ Enterocolitica /en' tero koli tica/ Bacteria causes Acute Enterocolitis with fever, abdominal pain and diarrhea.

The Yersinia /yersin' e a/ Enterocolitica /en' tero koli tica/ Bacteria is a Catalase Positive Enteric Bacteria.

The Yersinia /yersin' e a/ Enterocolitica /en' tero koli tica/ Bacteria is transmitted via contaminated food or water and unpasteurized milk.

The Yersinia /yersin' e a/ Enterocolitica /en' tero koli tica/ Bacteria has V and W antigens and motile virulence factors.

The Yersinia /yersin' e a/ Enterocolitica /en' tero koli tica/ Bacteria is treated with antibiotics even though they do not alter the course of the diarrhea.

Vibrio Cholera Bacteria

The Vibrio /vib' re o/ Cholera /kol' era/ Bacteria causes Chlorea with severe diarrhea.

The Vibrio /vib' re o/ Cholera /kol' era/ Bacteria is an Oxidase-Positive Vibrionaceae /vib' re on e a' si e/ Bacteria.

The Vibrio /vib' re o/ Cholera /kol' era/ Bacteria is transmitted via feces and orally.

The Vibrio /vib' re o/ Cholera /kol' era/ Bacteria expresses the following virulence factors; it is motile, muccinase, fimbriae, and noninvasive.

The Vibrio /vib' re o/ Cholera /kol' era/ Bacteria is treated with fluid replacement, Doxycycline and Fluoroquinolone.

Vibrio Parahaemolyticus Bacteria

The Vibrio /vib' re o/ Parahaemolyticus /per' ahe' molit' ikus/ Bacteria is the cause of 25% of the food poisoning in Japan. Symptoms include severe diarrhea that lasts for three days.

The Vibrio /vib' re o/ Parahaemolyticus /per' ahe' molit' ikus/ Bacteria is a Halophillic /halo' filik/ Vibrionaceae /vib' re on e a' si e/ Bacteria.

The Vibrio /vib' re o/ Parahaemolyticus /per' ahe' molit' ikus/ Bacteria is transmitted via of raw fish.

The Vibrio /vib' re o/ Parahaemolyticus /per' ahe' molit' ikus/ Bacteria has a motile H Angtigen and capsule virulence factors.

The Vibrio */vib' re o/* Parahaemolyticus */per' ahe' molit' ikus/* Bacteria is treated with Doxycycline and Fluoroquinolone.

Campylobacter Jejuni Bacteria

The Campylobacter */kamp' lo bak' ter/* Jejuni */jij' oone/* Bacteria causes bloody diarrhea.

The Campylobacter */kamp' lo bak' ter/* Jejuni */jij' oone/* is a Microaerophilic */mikro aro filik/* Oxidase Positive Vibrionaceae */vib' re on e a' si e/* Bacteria.

The Campylobacter */kamp' lo bak' ter/* Jejuni */jij' oone/* is transmitted via uncooked meat, unpasteurized milk, feces, orally.

The Campylobacter */kamp' lo bak' ter/* Jejuni */jij' oone/* has the following virulence factors; it is motile H-Antigen and invasive.

The Campylobacter */kamp' lo bak' ter/* Jejuni */jij' oone/* is treated with Fluoroquinolone and Erythromycin.

Helicobacter Pylori Bacteria

The Helicobacter */hel' iko bak' ter/* Pylori */pilor e/* Bacteria causes Duodenal Ulcers and Chronic Gastritis.

The Helicobacter */hel' iko bak' ter/* Pylori */pilor e/* Bacteria is a Microaerophillic */mikro aro filik/* Urease-Positive Vibrionaceae */vib' re on e a' si e/* Bacteria.

The Helicobacter /*hel' iko bak' ter*/ Pylori /*pilor e*/ Bacteria is treated with Bismuth, Ampicillin, Metronidazole and Tetracycline.

Pseudomonas Aeruginosa Bacteria

The Pseudomonas /*soodom' onas*/ Aeruginosa /*ar' ugin osa*/ Bacteria causes Pneumonia, Osteomyelitis, burn wound infections, Sepsis, urinary tract infections, Endocarditis, malignant external Otitis and corneal infections in individuals that wear contact lenses.

The Pseudomonas /*soodom' onas*/ Aeruginosa /*ar' ugin osa*/ Bacteria is an Obligate Aerobe Oxidase Positive Pseudomonadaceae /*soodom' ona e a' si e*/ Bacteria.

The Pseudomonas /*soodom' onas*/ Aeruginosa /*ar' ugin osa*/ Bacteria is treated with Ticarcillin, Timentin, Carbenicillin, Piperacillin, Mezlocillin, Ciprofloxacin, Imipenhem, Tobramycin, and Aztreonam.

Pseudomonas Cepacea Bacteria

The Pseudomonas /*soodom' onas*/ Cepacea /*sep' asea*/ Bacteria causes hospital acquired infections. It is extremely antibiotic and disinfectant resistant.

The Pseudomonas /*soodom' onas*/ Cepacea /*sep' asea* Bacteria is a Oxidase-Negative Pseudomonadaceae /*soodom' ona e a' si e*/ Bacteria.

The Pseudomonas /*soodom' onas*/ Cepacea /*sep' asea* Bacteria is treated with Trimethoprim combined with Sulfamethoxazole and Ciprofloxacin.

Xanthomonas Maltophilia Bacteria

The Xanthomonas /zan' thomon' as/ Maltophilia /mal' to fila/ Bacteria causes Pneumonia, Endocarditis and Meningitis.

The Xanthomonas /zan' thomon' as/ Maltophilia /mal' to fila/ Bacteria is an Oxidase-Negative Pseudomonadaceae /soodom' mna e a' si e/ Bacteria.

The Xanthomonas /zan' thomon' as/ Maltophilia /mal' to fila/ Bacteria is treated with Trimethoprim combined with Sulfamethoxazole and Ciprofloxacin.

Bacteroides Fragilis Bacteria

The Bacteroides /bak' tiroi' dez/ Fragilis /fraj' ilis/ Bacteria causes abscesses in the gastrointestinal tract, pelvis and legs.

The Bacteroides /bak' tiroi' dez/ Fragilis /fraj' ilis/ Bacteria is an Anerobic Gram-Positive Rod Bacteroidaceae /bak' tiroi' de a' si e/ Bacteria.

The Bacteroides /bak' tiroi' dez/ Fragilis /fraj' ilis/ Bacteria is found as part of the normal flora in the intestine.

The Bacteroides /bak' tiroi' dez/ Fragilis /fraj' ilis/ Bacteria is treated with Metronidazole, Clindamycin, and Chloramphenicol. A prevention measure is to surgically drain the abcesses.

Bacteroides Melaninogenicus Bacteria

The Bacteroides /bak' tiroi' dez/ Melaninogenicus /mel' a nino jen ikus/ Bacteria causes Necrotizing Anaerobic Pneumonia and Periodontal Disease.

The Bacteroides /*bak' tiroi' dez*/ Melaninogenicus /*mel' a nino jen ikus*/ Bacteria is an Anaerobic Gram-Positive Rod Bacteroidaceae /*bak' tiroi' de a' si e*/ Bacteria.

The Bacteroides /*bak' tiroi' dez*/ Melaninogenicus /*mel' a nino jen ikus*/ Bacteria is found as part of the normal flora in the intestine.

The Bacteroides /*bak' tiroi' dez*/ Melaninogenicus /*mel' a nino jen ikus*/ Bacteria is treated with Metronidazole and Clindamycin.

Fusobacterium Bacteria

The Fusobacterium /*fyoo' zho bak' ter um*/ Bacteria causes Necrotizing Anaerobic Pneumonia, Periodonatal Disease, abdominal and pelvic abscesses and Otitis Media.

The Fusobacterium /*fyoo' zho bak' ter um*/ Bacteria is an Anaerobic Gram-Negative Rod Bacteroidaceae /*bak' tiroi' de a' si e*/ Bacteria.

The Fusobacterium /*fyoo' zho bak' ter um*/ Bacteria is treated with Penicillin G.

Haemophilus Influenza Bacteria

The Haemophilus /*hemof' ilis*/ Influenza Bacteria causes Meningitis, Acute Epiglottitis, Septic Arthritis in infants, Sepsis, and Pneumonia.

The Haemophilus /*hemof' ilis*/ Influenza Bacteria is a

Haemophilus /*hemof' ilis*/ Gram Negative Rod Bacteria.

The Haemophilus /*hemof' ilis*/ Influenza Bacteria has the following virulence factors; 6 types of capsule, attachment pill and IgA1 protase.

The Haemophilus /*hemof' ilis*/ Influenza Bacteria is treated with second or third generation cephalosporins. Prevention is obtained from Hib Vaccine or via passive immunization where the mother is immunized during the 8th month of pregnancy to increase the antibody transfer in breast milk.

Haemophilus Ducreyi Bacteria

The Haemophilus /*hemof' ilis*/ Ducreyi /*duk' rei*/ Bacteria causes Chancroid, which includes symptoms of painful genital ulcer and swollen lymph nodes.

The Haemophilus /*hemof' ilis*/ Ducreyi /*duk' rei*/ Bacteria is a Haemophilus /*hemof' ilis*/ Gram Negative Rod Bacteria.

The Haemophilus /*hemof' ilis*/ Ducreyi /*duk' rei*/ Bacteria is sexually transmitted.

The Haemophilus /*hemof' ilis*/ Ducreyi /*duk' rei*/ Bacteria is treated with Azithromycin or erythromycin, Ceftriaxone, and Ciprofloxacin.

Gardnerella Vaginalis Bacteria

The Gardnerella /*gard' nerel' a*/ Vaginalis /*vaj' in alis*/ Bacteria causes Bacterial Vaginitis.

The Gardnerella /gard' nerel' a/ Vaginalis /vaj' in alis/ Bacteria is a Haemophilus /hemof' ilus/ Gram Negative Rod Bacteria.

The Gardnerella /gard' nerel' a/ Vaginalis /vaj' in alis/ Bacteria is sexually transmitted.

The Gardnerella /gard' nerel' a/ Vaginalis /vaj' in alis/ Bacteria has a no capsule virulence.

The Gardnerella /gard' nerel' a/ Vaginalis /vaj' in alis/ Bacteria is treated with Metronidazole.

Bordetella Pertussis Bacteria

The Bordetella /bor' ditel' a/ Pertussis /pertus' is/ Bacteria causes Whooping Cough.

The Bordetella /bor' ditel' a/ Pertussis /pertus' is/ Bacteria is transmitted via the respiratory system and is highly contagious.

The Bordetella /bor' ditel' a/ Pertussis /pertus' is/ Bacteria is a Bordetella /bor' ditel' a/ Gram Negative Rod Bacteria.

The Bordetella /bor' ditel' a/ Pertussis /pertus' is/ Bacteria has the following virulence factors; capsule, Beta-latamase, and Filamentous hemagglutinin.

The Bordetella /bor' ditel' a/ Pertussis /pertus' is/ Bacteria is treated with Erythromycin. The DPT vaccine offers prevention to this bacteria.

Legionella Pneumophila Bacteria

The Legionella /le' jinel' a/ Pneumophila /noomof' ila/ Bacteria causes Pontiac Fever and Legionnaires' Disease.

The Legionella /le' jinel' a/ Pneumophila /noomof' ila/ Bacteria is transmitted via air conditioning systems and cooling towers.

The Legionella /le' jinel' a/ Pneumophila /noomof' ila/ Bacteria is a Legionella /le' jinel' a/ gram negative rod bacteria.

The Legionella /le' jinel' a/ Pneumophila /noomof' ila/ Bacteria has the following virulence factors; capsule, motile, and hemolysin.

The Legionella /le' jinel' a/ Pneumophila /noomof' ila/ Bacteria is treated with Erythromycin and Rifampin.

Yersinia Pestis Bacteria

The Yersinia /yersin' e a/ Pestis /pest' is/ Bacteria causes Bubonic Plague, Sepsis, and Pneumonic Plague.

The Yersinia /yersin' e a/ Pestis /pest' is/ Bacteria is transmitted via infected fleas from wild rodents, city rats, and squirrels and prairie dogs in the South Western United States.

The Yersinia /yersin' e a/ Pestis /pest' is/ Bacteria is a Facultative Anaerobe Zoonotic Gram-Negative Rod Bacteria.

The Yersinia /yersin' e a/ Pestis /pest' is/ Bacteria has the following virulence factors; fraction 1 (F1), V and W proteins, and non-motile.

The Yersinia /*yersin' e a*/ Pestis /*pest' is*/ Bacteria is treated with Streptomycin or Gentamicin, and Doxycycline. There is a killed vaccine that is effective for a few months. The attenuated vaccine is more effective but also has more side effects.

Yerisinia Enterocolitica Bacteria

The Yerisinia /*yersin' e a*/ Enterocolitica /*en' terok o litika*/ Bacteria causes Enterocolitis, Arthritis and a rash.

The Yerisinia /*yersin' e a*/ Enterocolitica /*en' terok o litika*/ Bacteria is transmitted via unpasteurized milk.

The Yerisinia /*yersin' e a*/ Enterocolitica /*en' terok o litika*/ Bacteria is a Facultative Anaerobe Zoonotic Gram-Negative Rod Bacteria.

The Yerisinia /*yersin' e a*/ Enterocolitica /*en' terok o litika*/ Bacteria has the following virulence factors; invasive, V and W proteins, and motile at 25 degrees Celsius.

The Yerisinia /*yersin' e a*/ Enterocolitica /*en' terok o litika*/ Bacteria is treated with Fluoroquinolone and Trimethoprim/Sulfamethoxazole.

Francisella Tularensis Bacteria

The Francisella /*fran' si' sela*/ Tularensis /*tu' lar en' sis*/ Bacteria causes Tularemia with symptoms of ulceroglandular at the site of the tick bite or direct contact with contaminated rabbit, pneumonia, oculoglandular and typhoidal.

The Francisella /*fran' si' sela*/ Tularensis /*tu' lar en' sis*/ Bacteria is transmitted via ticks that have been on infected rabbits and squirrels. The transmission comes from a bite, direct contact with infected animal tissue, inhaled aerosolized organisms, or ingestion of contaminated meat or water.

The Francisella /*fran' si' sela*/ Tularensis /*tu' lar en' sis*/ Bacteria is an Obligate Aerobe Zoonotic Gram-Negative Rod Bacteria.

The Francisella /*fran' si' sela*/ Tularensis /*tu' lar en' sis*/ Bacteria has a non-motile capsule virulence factor.

The Francisella /*fran' si' sela*/ Tularensis /*tu' lar en' sis*/ Bacteria is treated with Gentamicin or Streptomycin, Doxycycline. There is a attenuated vaccine that is currently available for high risk individuals only.

Brucella Melitensis Bacteria

The Brucella /*broo' sela*/ Melitensis /*mel' iten sis*/ Bacteria causes Brucellosis that results in fluctuating fever, weakness and loss of appetite.

The Brucella /*broo' sela*/ Melitensis /*mel' iten sis*/ Bacteria is transmitted via direct contact with infected goats or aborted goat placentas. It can also be transmitted through contaminated milk.

The Brucella /*broo' sela*/ Melitensis /*mel' iten sis*/ Bacteria is an Obligate Aerobe Zoonotic Gram Negative Rod Brucella Bacteria.

The Brucella /broo' sela/ Melitensis /mel' iten sis/ Bacteria has the following virulence factors; capsule, non-motile, and Tropism for erythritol.

The Brucella /broo' sela/ Melitensis /mel' iten sis/ Bacteria is treated with a combination of Doxycycline and Gentamicin. The Brucella Melitensis Bacteria is prevented through pasteurization of milk and immunization of cattle.

Pasterurella Multocida Bacteria

The Pasterurella /pas' terul' la/ Multocida /multo' sida/ Bacteria causes wound infections following dog or cat bites.

The Pasterurella /pas' terul' la/ Multocida /multo' sida/ Bacteria is transmitted via dog and cat bites. The bacteria is found naturally in domestic and wild animals.

The Pasterurella /pas' terul' la/ Multocida /multo' sida/ Bacteria is a Facultative Anaerobe Zoonotic Gram Negative Bacteria.

The Pasterurella /pas' terul' la/ Multocida /multo' sida/ Bacteria has the following virulence factors; capsule and non-motile.

The Pasterurella /pas' terul' la/ Multocida /multo' sida/ Bacteria is treated with Penicillin G, Doxycycline, and third generation Cephalosporin.

Treponema Pallidum Bacteria

The Treponema /trep' one' ma/ Pallidum /pal' i dum/ Bacteria causes Syphilis.

The Treponema /trep' one' ma/ Pallidum /pal' i dum/ Bacteria is transmitted sexually between humans.

The Treponema /trep' one' ma/ Pallidum /pal' i dum/ Bacteria is a Spirochete /spi' ro' ket/ Gram Negative Bacteria.

The Treponema /trep' one' ma/ Pallidum /pal' i dum/ Bacteria virulence factor is motile.

The Treponema /trep' one' ma/ Pallidum /pal' i dum/ Bacteria is treated with Penicillin G, Erythromycin and Doxycycline.

Treponema Pallidum Bacteria subspecies endemicum

The Treponema /trep' one' ma/ Pallidum /pal' i dum/ Bacteria causes Bejel.

The Treponema /trep' one' ma/ Pallidum /pal' i dum/ Bacteria is transmitted via sharing food or drink and contaminated eating utensils.

The Treponema /trep' one' ma/ Pallidum /pal' i dum/ Bacteria is a Spirochete /spi ro' ket/ Gram Negative Bacteria.

The Treponema /trep' one' ma/ Pallidum /pal' i dum/ Bacteria virulence factor is motile.

The Treponema /trep' one' ma/ Pallidum /pal' i dum/ Bacteria is treated with Penicillin.

Treponema Pertenue Bacteria

The Treponema */trep' one' ma/* Pertenue */per' ten u/* Bacteria causes Yaws which is skin lesions.

The Treponema */trep' one' ma/* Pertenue */per' ten u/* Bacteria is transmitted via direct contact or via infected flies.

The Treponema */trep' one' ma/* Pertenue */per' ten u/* Bacteria is a Spirochete */spi ro' ket/* Gram Negative Bacteria.

The Treponema */trep' one' ma/* Pertenue */per' ten u/* Bacteria virulence factor is motile.

The Treponema */trep' one' ma/* Pertenue */per' ten u/* Bacteria is treated with Penicillin and plastic surgery for correction of facial disfigurement.

Treponema Carateum Bacteria

The Treponema */trep' one' ma/* Carateum /kar at um/ Bacteria causes Pinta which is flat red or blue lesions that do not ulcerate.

The Treponema */trep' one' ma/* Carateum /kar at um/ Bacteria is transmitted via direct contact.

The Treponema */trep' one' ma/* Carateum /kar at um/ Bacteria is a Spirochete */spi ro' ket/* Gram Negative Bacteria.

The Treponema */trep' one' ma/* Carateum /kar at um/ Bacteria virulence factor is motile.

The Treponema */trep' one' ma/* Carateum /kar at um/ Bacteria is treated with Penicillin.

Borrelia Burgdorferi Bacteria

The Borrelia /*borel' e a*/ Burgdorferi /*burg' dorfer' i*/ Bacteria causes Lyme Disease.

The Borrelia /*borel' e a*/ Burgdorferi /*burg' dorfer' i*/ Bacteria is transmitted via ticks from the white-footed mouse or the white-tailed deer.

The Borrelia /*borel' e a*/ Burgdorferi /*burg' dorfer' i*/ Bacteria is a Spirochete /*spi ro' ket*/ Gram Negative Bacteria.

The Borrelia /*borel' e a*/ Burgdorferi /*burg' dorfer' i*/ Bacteria is treated with Doxycycline, Amoxicillan, and Ceftriaxone for neurologic disease.

Additional Species of Borrelia Bacteria

The 18 additional species of Borrelia /*borel' e a*/ Bacteria cause relapsing fever and occasional rash.

The 18 additional species of Borrelia /*borel' e a*/ Bacteria are transmitted via vectors that have been infected from wild rodents.

The 18 additional species of Borrelia /*borel' e a*/ Bacteria are Spirochete /*spi ro' ket*/ Gram Negative Bacteria.

The 18 additional species of Borrelia /*borel' e a*/ Bacteria are treated with Doxycycline, Erythromycin, Penicillin G.

Leptospira Interrogans Bacteria

The Leptospira /*lep' to spi' ra*/ Interrogans /*in' terog' ans*/ Bacteria cause organisms in the blood and high spiking temperatures. This can progress into the second phase which includes the above symptoms with severe neck pain. In severe cases it can develop into Weil's Disease.

The Leptospira /lep' to spi' ra/ Interrogans /in' terog' ans/ Bacteria is transmitted via direct contact with infected urine or animal tissue of infected animals.

The Leptospira /lep' to spi' ra/ Interrogans /in' terog' ans/ Bacteria are Spirochete /spi ro' ket/ Gram Negative Bacteria.

The Leptospira /lep' to spi' ra/ Interrogans /in' terog' ans/ Bacteria are treated with Penicillin G and Doxycycline.

Mycobacterium Tuberculosis Bacteria

The Mycobacterium /mi' kobaktir' e um/ Tuberculosis /tyoobur' kyulo' sis/ Bacteria cause Tuberculosis.

The Mycobacterium /mi' kobaktir' e um/ Tuberculosis /tyoobur' kyulo' sis/ Bacteria is an Aerobic Catalase Positive Mycobacterium /mi' kobaktir' e um/ Bacteria.

The Mycobacterium /mi' kobaktir' e um/ Tuberculosis /tyoobur' kyulo' sis/ Bacteria the virulence factors include; Mycosides, Sulfatides, Wax D, Iron Siderophore, and facultative intracellular growth.

The Mycobacterium /mi' kobaktir' e um/ Tuberculosis /tyoobur' kyulo' sis/ Bacteria is treated with Isoniazid, Rifampin, Pyrazinamide, Ethambutol, and Streptomycin.

Mycobacterium Leprae Bacteria

The Mycobacterium /mi' kobaktir' e um/ Leprae /lep' ra/ Bacteria causes Leprosy.

The Mycobacterium /mi' kobaktir' e um/ Leprae /lep' ra/ Bacteria is a Catalase Positive Mycobacterium /mi' kobaktir' e um/ Bacteria.

The Mycobacterium /mi' kobaktir' e um/ Leprae /lep' ra/ Bacteria has the following virulence factors; non-motile and facultative intracellular growth.

The Mycobacterium /mi' kobaktir' e um/ Leprae /lep' ra/ Bacteria is treated with Rifampin, Dapsone, and Clofazimine.

Mycoplasma Pneumonia Bacteria

The Mycoplasma /mi' koplaz' ma/ Pneumonia Bacteria causes Tracheobronchitis and Walking Pneumonia.

The Mycoplasma /mi' koplaz' ma/ Pneumonia Bacteria is a Facultative Anaerobe Mycoplasma Bacteria.

The Mycoplasma /mi' koplaz' ma/ Pneumonia Bacteria has a protein P1 virulence factor.

The Mycoplasma /mi' koplaz' ma/ Pneumonia Bacteria is treated with Erythromycin and Tetracycline.

Ureaplasma Urealyticum Bacteria

The Ureaplasma /yoor' e plaz' ma/ Urealyticum /yoor' e litikum/ Bacteria causes Non-Gonococcal Urethritis.

The Ureaplasma */yoor' e plaz' ma/* Urealyticum */yoor' e litikum/* Bacteria is a Urease Mycoplasma Bacteria.

The Ureaplasma */yoor' e plaz' ma/* Urealyticum */yoor' e litikum/* Bacteria is treated with Erythromycin and Tetracycline.

Actinomyces Israelii Bacteria

The Actinomyces */ak' tinomi' sez/* Israelii */iz ra' le/* Bacteria causes eroding abcesses of the mouth, lung or gastrointestinal tract.

The Actinomyces */ak' tinomi' sez/* Israelii */iz ra' le/* Bacteria is an Acid Fast Gram Positive Anaerobic Bacteria. It is found in the normal flora of the gastrointestinal tract and the mouth.

The Actinomyces */ak' tinomi' sez/* Israelii */iz ra' le/* Bacteria is treated with Penicillin G and surgery.

Nocardia Asteroides Bacteria

The Nocardia */nokar' dea/* Asteroides */as' te roidz/* Bacteria causes Pneumonia and formation of abcesses in the lung, kidney and central nervous system.

The Nocardia */nokar' dea/* Asteroides */as' te roidz/* Bacteria is an Acid Fast Gram Positive Aerobic Bacteria.

The Nocardia */nokar' dea/* Asteroides */as' te roidz/* Bacteria is treated with Trimethoprim/Sulfamethoxazole.

Fungi

Fungi are eucaryotic cells that do not contain chlorophyll. Fungi require an aerobic environment.

Malassezia Furfur Fungi

The Malassezia /mal' ase' ze a/ Furfur /fur' fur/ Fungi causes Pityriasis Veraicolor. Symptoms include discolored light patches on the skin.

The Malassezia /mal' ase' ze a/ Furfur /fur' fur/ Fungi is a Hyphae Spherical Yeast Fungus that causes superficial fungal infections.

Covering the affected area with dandruff shampoo containing Selenium Sulfide treats the MMalassezia /mal' ase' ze a/ Furfur /fur' fur/ Fungi.

Exophiala Wermeckii Fungi

The Exophiala /ek' sofil'a/ Wemeckii /wem' eke/ Fungi causes Tinea Nigra. Symptoms include dark brown patches on the soles of the hands and feet.

The Exophiala /ek' sofil'a/ Wemeckii /wem' eke/ Fungi is a Hyphae Spherical Yeast Fungus that causes superficial fungal infections.

Covering the affected area with dandruff shampoo containing Selenium Sulfide treats the Exophiala /ek' sofil'a/ Wemeckii

/wem' eke/ Fungi.

Microsporum Fungi

The Microsporum /mi' kro spo' rum/ Fungi causes Ring Worm, Jock Itch, Athlete's Foot, Tinea Capitis of the scalp, and Onychomycosis.

The Microsporum /mi' kro spo' rum/ Fungi is a Dermatophyte Fungus that causes cutaneous fungal infections. The Microsporum fungus is found in the soil.

The Microsporum /mi' kro spo' rum/ Fungi is treated with a Topical Imidazole, oral Griseofulvin, and oral Terminafine.

Trichophyton Fungi

The Trichophyton /trik' o fitun/ Fungi causes Ring Worm, Jock Itch, Athlete's Foot, Tinea Capitis of the scalp, and Onychomycosis.

The Trichophyton /trik' o fitun/ Fungi is a Dermatophyte Fungus that causes cutaneous fungal infections. The Microsporum fungus is found on animals.

The Trichophyton /trik' o fitun/ Fungi is treated with a Topical Imidazole, oral Griseofulvin, and oral Terminafine.

Epidermophyton Floccosum Fungi

The Epidermophyton /ep' idur' mofiton/ Floccosum /flok' osum/ Fungi causes Ring Worm, Jock Itch, Athlete's Foot, Tinea Capitis of the scalp, and Onychomycosis.

The Epidermophyton /ep' idur' mofiton/ Floccosum /flok' osum/ Fungi is a Dermatophyte Fungus that causes cutaneous fungal infections. The Microsporum fungus resides on humans.

The Epidermophyton /ep' idur' mofiton/ Floccosum /flok' osum/ Fungi is treated with a Topical Imidazole, oral Griseofulvin, and Oral Terminafine.

Sporothrix Schenckii Fungi

The Sporothrix /spor' o triks/ Schenckii /shen' ki/ Fungi causes Sporotrichosis. The symptoms include a raised ulcerating nodule that will appear at the puncture site of the rose thorn . The initial nodule will heal, but additional nodules will appear along the same lymphatic tract.

The Sporothrix /spor' o triks/ Schenckii /shen' ki/ Fungi is a Dimorphic Fungi commonly found in soil and on plants that causes subcutaneous fungal infections.

The Sporothrix /spor' o triks/ Schenckii /shen' ki/ Fungi is treated with oral Potassium Iodide, Amphotericin B, and Itraconazole.

Phialophora Verrucosa Fungi

The Phialophora /fil' ofor a/ Verrucosa /veroo' kosa/ Fungi causes Chromoblastomycosis. Symptoms include a small violet wart-like lesion that develops after a puncture wound. Over time, small clusters of these lesions can develop to resemble cauliflower.

The Phialophora /fil' ofor a/ Verrucosa /veroo' kosa/ Fungi is a copper colored soil Phialophora and Cladosporium Saprophyte Fungi that is usually found on rotting wood.

The Phialophora /fil' ofor a/ Verrucosa /veroo' kosa/ Fungi is treated with Itraconazole and local excision.

Cladosporium Carrionii Fungi

The Cladosporium /klad' o spori' um/ Carrionii /kar' eone/ Fungi causes Chromoblastomycosis. Symptoms include a small violet wart-like lesion that develops after a puncture wound. Over time, small clusters of these lesions can develop to resemble cauliflower.

The Cladosporium /klad' o spori' um/ Carrionii /kar' eone/ Fungi is a copper colored soil Phialophora and Cladosporium Saprophyte Fungi that is usually found on rotting wood.

The Cladosporium /klad' o spori' um/ Carrionii /kar' eone/ Fungi is treated with Itraconazole and local excision.

Fonsecaea Fungi

The Fonsecaea /fon' seke/ Fungi causes Chromoblastomycosis. Symptoms include a small violet wart-like lesion that develops after a puncture wound. Over time, small clusters of these lesions can develop to resemble cauliflower.

The Fonsecaea /fon' seke/ Fungi is a copper colored soil Phialophora and Cladosporium Saprophyte Fungi that is usually found on rotting wood.

The Fonsecaea /*fon' seke*/ Fungi is treated with Itraconazole and local excision.

Coccidioides Immitis Fungi

The Coccidioides /*kosid' e oids*/ Immitis /*im' itus*/ Fungi causes Coccidioidomycosis. This is asymptomatic infection that can cause Pneumonia.

The Coccidioides /*kosid' e oids*/ Immitis /*im' itus*/ Fungi is Dimorphic Mycelial and Yeast fungi that is transmiited via the respiratory system.

The Coccidioides /*kosid' e oids*/ Immitis /*im' itus*/ Fungi is treated with Amphotericicin B, Itraconazole, and Fluconazole.

Histoplasma Capsulatum Fungi

The Histoplasma /*his' to plaz' ma*/ Capsulatum /*kap' sy' latam*/ Fungi causes Histoplasmosis. This is an asymptomatic infection that can cause Pnemonia with lesions that calcify and it can spread to other organs of the body.

The Histoplasma /*his' to plaz' ma*/ Capsulatum /*kap' sy' latam*/ Fungi is Dimorphic Mycelial and Yeast fungi that is spread via bird and rat droppings and respiratory transmission.

The Histoplasma /*his' to plaz' ma*/ Capsulatum /*kap' sy' latam*/ Fungi is treated with Itraconazole and Ammphotericin B.

Blastomyces Dermatitidis Fungi

The Blastomyces /*blas' tomi' sez*/ Dermatitidis /*dur' mati dis*/ Fungi causes Blastomycosis. Symptoms include pneumonia with lesions that rarely calcify, skin ulcers, weight loss, and night sweats.

The Blastomyces /blas' tomi' sez/ Dermatitidis /dur' mati dis/ Fungi is a Dimorphic Mycelial and Yeast Fungi that is resides in the soil and rotten wood in the Mississippi River Valley.

The Blastomyces /blas' tomi' sez/ Dermatitidis /dur' mati dis/ Fungi is treated with Itraconazole, Ketoconazole, and Amphotericin B.

Cryptococcus Neoformans Fungi

Cryptococcus /krip' to kokus/ Neoformans /ne for' manz/ Fungi causes Cryptococcosis. Symptoms include subacute or chronic Meningitis, Pneumonia and skin lesions that resemble acne.

Cryptococcus /krip' to kokus/ Neoformans /ne for' manz/ Fungi is a Polysaccharide Capsule Yeast form fungi that is found in pigeon droppings.

Cryptococcus /krip' to kokus/ Neoformans /ne for' manz/ Fungi is treated with Amphotericin B, Flucytosine and Fluconazole.

Candida Albicans Fungi

The Candida /kan' dida/ Albicans /al' bikanz/ Fungi causes oral thrush, Vulvovaginal Candidiasis, diaper rash and rash in the skin folds of obese persons.

The Candida /kan' dida/ Albicans /al' bikanz/ Fungi is a Pseudohyphae and Yeast Fungi.

The Candida /kan' dida/ Albicans /al' bikanz/ Fungi is treated with Nystatin or Imidazole candies for oral thrush, and Topical Imidazole for cutaneous infections.

Aspergillus Fumigatus Fungi

The Aspergillus /as' perjil' us/ Fumigatus /fyoo' miga tus/ Fungi causes Allergic Bronchopulmonary Aspergillosis which is an asthma type reaction.

The Aspergillus /as' perjil' us/ Fumigatus /fyoo' miga tus/ Fungi is a Branching Septated Hyphae Aspergillus Fungi.

The Aspergillus /as' perjil' us/ Fumigatus /fyoo' miga tus/ Fungi is treated with Corticosteroids.

Aspergillus Flavus Fungi

The Aspergillus /as' perjil' us/ Flavus /flav' us/ Fungi causes Aspergilloma which is a fungus ball that is associated with a bloody cough.

The Aspergillus /as' perjil' us/ Flavus /flav' us/ Fungi is a Branching Septated Hyphae Aspergillus Fungi.

Removing it via surgery treats the Aspergillus /as' perjil' us/ Flavus /flav' us/ Fungi.

Aspergillus Niger Fungi

The Aspergillus /as' perjil' us/ Niger /nij' er/ Fungi causes Invasive Aspergillosis which is a Necrotizing Pneumonia.

The Aspergillus /as' perjil' us/ Niger /nij' er/ Fungi is a Branching Septated Hyphae Aspergillus Fungi.

The Aspergillus /as' perjil' us/ Niger /nij' er/ Fungi is treated with Amphotericin B.

References

Gladwin, M., Trattler, B., Clinical Microbiology Made Ridiculously Simple 2nd edition, Medmaster, Inc.

Chamberlain, N., Medical Microbiology: Neal Chamberlain's Look at Microbes

Barron, S., Medical Microbiology Textbook, University of Texas Medical Branch

Anderson, K., Mosby's Pocket Dictionary of Medicine, Nursing & Allied Health, 3rd Edition, Mosby

Costello, R., Random House Webster's College Dictionary

You have reached the end of the audio review for
Medical Microbiology.

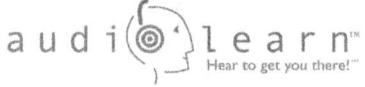

www.ingramcontent.com/pod-product-compliance
Lightning Source LLC
Chambersburg PA
CBHW070930180526
45168CB00003B/1013